Labour Midwifery Skills

Survival Guide

2nd Edition

Alison Edwards

T0156165

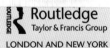

Routledge
Taylor & Francis Group

LONDON AND NEW YORK

Second edition published 2021
by Routledge
2 Park Square, Milton Park, Abingdon, Oxon, OX14 4RN

and by Routledge
52 Vanderbilt Avenue, New York, NY 10017

Routledge is an imprint of the Taylor & Francis Group, an informa business

First edition published by Pearson Education Limited 2012

British Library Cataloguing-in-Publication Data
A catalogue record for this book is available from the British Library

Library of Congress Cataloging-in-Publication Data
A catalog record has been requested for this book

ISBN: 978-1-138-38889-5 (pbk)
ISBN: 978-0-429-42429-8 (ebk)

Typeset in Helvetica
by Cenveo® Publisher Services

contents

Figures

Tables

Abbreviations

TIP

Many abbreviations are used in midwifery; however, officially *only those accepted by your individual Trust should be used.*

APH	ante-partum haemorrhage
ARM	artificial rupture of membranes
BD	twice daily
BMI	body mass index
BP	blood pressure
BPM	beats per minute
C/O	care of/complaining of
CAF	Common Assessment Framework
CCT	controlled cord traction
CRL	crown rump length
CTG	cardiotocograph
DOB	date of birth
DV	domestic violence
DVT	deep vein thrombosis
EBL	Estimated blood loss
ECV	external cephalic version
EDD	estimated due date/estimated date of delivery
FBC	fluid balance chart or full blood count

FBS	fetal blood sample
FD	forceps delivery
FGM	female genital mutilation
FH	fundal height
FHHR	fetal heart heard and regular/reactive
FL	femur length
FM	fetal movements
FSE	fetal scalp electrode
G	gravida (the number of pregnancies)
G & S	group and save
H/O	history of
Hb	haemoglobin
HC	head circumference
HELLP	haemolysis, elevated liver enzymes and low platelets
HVS	high vaginal swab
IUCD	intrauterine contraceptive device
IUD	intrauterine death
IUGR	intrauterine growth restriction
IVI	Intravenous Infusion
LBW	low birthweight
LFT	liver function tests
LOA	left occipito anterior
LOP	left occipito posterior
LSCS	lower segment Caesarean section
MC & S	microscopy and sensitivity

MEW/MEOW	modified early (obstetric) warning score
ML	millilitre
MLC	midwifery-led care
MSU	mid-stream urine
NAD	no abnormalities detected
NBM	nil by mouth
NNU	neonatal unit
NVB	normal vaginal birth
OA	occipito anterior
OP	occipito posterior
P	parity (the number of births over 24 weeks)
PO	per oral
PR	per rectum
PV	per vagina
ROA	right occipito anterior
ROP	right occipito posterior
SB	stillbirth
SC	subcutaneous
SCBU	special care baby unit
SGA	small for gestational age
SOB	suboccipito-bregmatic
SROM	spontaneous rupture of membranes
TDS	three times daily
TPR	temperature, pulse and respirations

U & E	urea and electrolytes
USS	ultrasound scan
UTI	urinary tract infection
VBAC	vaginal birth after caesarean
VE	vaginal examination
Xmatch	cross-match

Anatomy

■ PELVIC FLOOR

A gutter-shaped structure which is higher anteriorly
than posteriorly. This aids rotation of the fetus during the
mechanism of labour.

Six layers:

1. Skin.
2. Fat.
3. Superficial muscles – transverse perinea, bulbocavernosa,
   ischiocavernosus. The urethral and anal sphincters are
   also found here.
4. Deep muscle layer – iliococcygeus, ischiococcygeus and
   the pubococcygeus.
5. Pelvic fascia which forms the pelvic ligaments.
6. Peritoneum.

The triangular perineal body consisting of the skin,
bulbocavernosus, transverse perinei and the pubococcygeus
assists with childbirth and defecation. It is these structures
which can stretch and tear, or are cut during an episiotomy
and require repair during childbirth.

■ PELVIS (GYNAECOID)

- *False pelvis* – the bony structures situated above the brim,
  which have no significance for childbearing.
- *True pelvis* – the structures found beneath the false pelvis,
  which form the birth canal. The ring of bones form the
  brim, cavity and outlet.

Bones

5 × fused sacral vertebrae make up the curved sacrum.
4 × fused vertebrae make up the coccyx.
2 × innominate bones – each of which consists of the ilium,
the ischium and a pubic bone. These bones meet at the
cup-shaped depression known as the acetabulum or hip
socket.

Joints

2 × sacroiliac joints which lie between the sacrum and the
ilium plus the symphysis pubis – a pad of cartilage between
the pubic bones.
    The sacrococcygeal joint – between the sacrum and
coccyx.

Ligaments

Sacrotuberous (from the sacrum to the ischial tuberosity) and
the sacrospinus (from the ischial spines to the sacrum). Both
of these ligaments form borders of the obstetric outlet.
    Different pelvic shapes – android, anthropoid and
platypelloid.

ACTIVITY

Consider how this structure helps with the mechanism of labour. Think about
positions for birth.

Table 1 Diameters of the gynaecoid pelvis

	DIAMETERS	SHAPE
Brim	Anterior–posterior = 11cm Oblique = 12cm Transverse = 13cm	Rounded
Cavity	All diameters are 12cm	Round
Obstetric outlet	Anterior–posterior = 13cm Oblique = 12cm Transverse = 11cm	Diamond

Figure 1 The gynaecoid pelvis

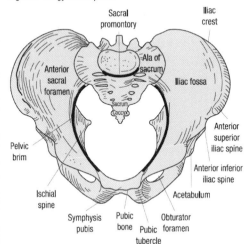

The landmarks of the brim

Think about these when defining fetal position.

Figure 2 Landmarks of the pelvic brim

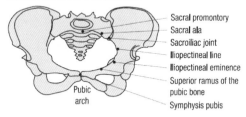

- Sacral promontory
- Sacral ala
- Sacroiliac joint
- Iliopectineal line
- Iliopectineal eminence
- Superior ramus of the pubic bone
- Symphysis pubis

Pubic arch

■ PLACENTA AND MEMBRANES

- Maternal side – consists of up to 22 cotyledons, made up of thousands of chorionic villi, separated by sulci.
- Fetal side – smooth and shiny and covered in membrane.
- Two membranes – the outer chorion, an opaque thin friable membrane, and the inner tough transparent amniotic membrane.
- Cord – consists of two arteries and one vein surrounded by Wharton's jelly. Twisted for strength. Most often attached to the centre of the placenta on the fetal side. Other forms of attachment include battledore and velamentous insertions.

Figure 3 Fetal and maternal sides of the placenta

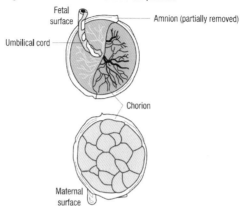

Figure 4 Diameters of the fetal skull

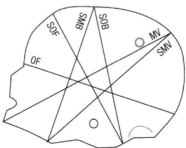

Table 2 Diameters of the fetal skull measurements

Suboccipito Bregmatic	9.5cm	Vertex (S.O.B.)	
Sub-occipitofrontal	10.0cm	Breech A.C.H (S.O.F.)	
Occipitofrontal	11.5cm	Face to pubis = P.O.P. (O.F.)	
Mentovertical	13.5cm	Brow (obstructed labour) (M.V.)	
Submentovertical	11.0cm	Face not fully extended (S.M.V.)	
Submento Bregmatic	9.5cm	Face fully extended (S.M.B.)	
Biparietal	9.5cm	Circumferences	S.O.B. 29.2cm
Bitemporal	8.3cm		O.F. 35.6cm
			M.V. 38.0cm

APGAR scores

- Undertaken at 1 minute, 5 minutes and 10 minutes following the birth.
- Scores out of 10.

Table 3 APGAR scores

	0	1	2
Heart rate	Absent	Below 100 beats/min	Over 100 beats/min
Respirations	Absent	Weak cry	Strong cry
Muscle tone	Limp	Some tone	Active motion
Reflex irritability	No response	Grimace	Cry
Colour	Blue or pale	Body pink, arms and legs blue	Completely pink

Birth environment – promoting normality

For extra ideas consider the midwifery care in labour guidance for all women in all settings. Blue top guidance no. 1 produced by the Royal College of Midwives (RCM 2018).

- Dim the lights – a relaxed mother will aid the release of natural oxytocin and endorphins.
- Maintain a comfortable room temperature – women are likely to get hot so find ways to cool them down (fans, cold flannels). *Remember* that the baby needs to be warm, so the room needs to be warm for the birth itself.
- Make the room less clinical – hide as much of the equipment as you can.
- Move the bed to a corner – don't make it the focus of the room.
- Encourage mobility – use mats, birthing balls, slings, upright positions. These will aid descent and rotation of the fetus during labour.
- Use water – for many women water is relaxing and soothing. This may be in a pool, bath or simply letting the warm water of a shower gently massage the lower back.
- Limit noise, interruptions and interventions – think: *do you need to do that VE?* However, having the woman's favourite music playing can also help.
- Complementary therapies such as aromatherapy, reflexology, hypnotherapy, massage and acupuncture. Depending on the type, appropriately trained staff may be needed. However, even a simple back massage can be helpful.
- Avoid setting rigid time limits for the labour as long as the woman and fetus are well.
- Avoid directed pushing during the second stage.

Blood values

Electrolytes

- Sodium (Na)   134–146mmol/L
- Potassium (K)   3.4–5.0mmol/L
- Glucose   3.0–7.8mmol/L
                                       3.9–6.2mmol/L (fasting)
- Urea (age-dependent)   4.0–8.0mmol/L
- Creatinine (age-dependent)   0.05–0.12mmol/L
- Total protein   63–78g/L
- Albumin   35–45g/L
- Globulin   25–45g/L
- Bilirubin total   3–17pmol/L
- Alkaline phosphatase (ALP)   35–150U/L
- Gamma GT   5–40U/L
- Alanine transaminase (ALT)   1–45U/L
- Aspartate transaminase (AST)   1–36U/L
- Calcium (Ca)   2.15–2.60mmol/L
- Total cholesterol   <200mg/dL
                                       <5.5mmol/L (fasting)

Blood gases

- pH   7.36–7.44
- pCO_2 36–44mmHg
- PaO_2 85–100mmHg
- Bicarbonate   22–29mmol/L
- Base excess   −2 to +2mmol/L
- Oxygen saturation   94–98%

Thyroid function tests

Thyroid-stimulating hormone (TSH) 1–11mU/L.

Haematology

- WBC $4.5–11 \times 10^9$/L
- RBC   Female $4.2–5.4 \times 10^9$/L
- Hb   Female 120–160g/L
- Mean cell volume (MCV)   80–100fL
- Platelets $150–400 \times 10^9$/L
- Lymphocytes   25–33%

Caesarean section (LSCS)

There are a number of approaches that can be used to categorise LSCS depending on the degree of urgency.

For example:

1. = **IMMEDIATE** – there is an immediate threat to the life of the woman or fetus (within 30 minutes of decision).
2. = **URGENT** – maternal or fetal compromise which is not immediately life-threatening but a significant delay could lead to an adverse outcome (within 30 to 75 minutes).
3. = **EMERGENCY NON-URGENT** – no maternal or fetal compromise, but needs early delivery (within 2 hours of decision).
4. = **ELECTIVE** – delivery preplanned around 39/40.

NICE (2019a).

■ PREPARATION

The urgency of the procedure will dictate the speed of preparation, but to ensure safety the woman should be as prepared as thoroughly as possible.

- Admit – take a full history and establish the reason for the lower segment Caesarean section (LSCS). Identify any allergies and apply a red alert wristband if there are any. Apply an identity wristband which should clearly state the woman's name, unit number, blood group and date of birth.
- Explain the procedure – what will happen before, during and afterwards.
- Ensure that a full blood count and group and save have been conducted. Check results. If appropriate request a cross-match (e.g. if the LSCS is for a Grade IV placenta praevia). Inform the medical team if the Hb or platelet level is low.

- Ensure that the woman has been nil by mouth for at least six hours – not always possible if, for example, there is a cord prolapse. Inform the anaesthetist if not.
- Administer any prescribed pre-operation medication (e.g. Ranitidine 150mg). 30ml of sodium citrate may also be given on transfer to theatre.
- Measure for and apply support stockings to reduce the risk of deep vein thrombosis (DVT).
- Change the woman into a gown – remove all underwear.
- Remove any jewelry, including tongue piercings. Wedding rings can be taped.
- Nail varnish should be removed.
- Removing the top inch of pubic hair is no longer recommended as this increases the infection risk; however, it can make removing any dressings more comfortable. Ideally, if a woman prefers to shave, this should be done 24 hours prior to the procedure to enable the skin surface to heal over.
- Following an abdominal examination, a cardiotocograph (CTG) can be conducted (depending on hospital policy). If the procedure is for a breech presentation a scan may also be conducted to confirm this.
- The woman should be seen by the anaesthetist and the obstetrician and consent for the procedure obtained.
- An indwelling catheter will need to be inserted. This can either be done in the privacy of the room or more commonly in theatre once the anaesthetic has been administered.
- Complete the required documentation – including the checklist, drug chart, fluid balance chart, pressure sore assessment, modified early obstetric warning score (MEOWS) and thromboembolic risk assessment sheet.

Catheterisation

■ PROCEDURE

- Obtain consent/ensure privacy.
- Wash hands.
- Collect equipment (catheter, drainage bag if required, catheter/vaginal examination [VE] pack, analgesic gel, sterile water or antiseptic lotion for cleansing, 10ml sterile water in a sterile syringe (if an indwelling catheter is required), sterile gloves and apron). Catheter bag stand if needed. Use a thoroughly cleaned trolley.
- Position the woman – semi-recumbent, ankles together, knees apart. Cover legs until procedure starts.
- Set up trolley with equipment. If an assistant is present, they can open the packaging and drop the contents onto your sterile field. If alone, open inner pack wearing sterile gloves, drop the remaining equipment onto the sterile field and then change gloves. Retain the catheter within the inner plastic wrapper.
- Ask the assistant or woman to lift the cover off her legs.
- Cleanse the vulval area – wipe top to bottom with each swab only once using the non-dominant hand. Place a sterile sheet under the woman's buttocks.
- With the non-dominant hand, part the labia and visualise the urethra.
- If used – insert the anaesthetic gel and wait for 3–5 minutes for this to take effect.
- Place the sterile receiver near the vulva and using the dominant hand insert the catheter. Gently advance the catheter until some urine is seen. Sterility is maintained by drawing back the plastic wrapper as the catheter is inserted.

- Once urine is seen, advance the catheter 3–5cm to ensure the balloon is fully in the bladder.
- Inflate the balloon using up to 10ml of the sterile water in the syringe. NB: some gentle pressure on the syringe plunger is needed when removing the syringe to avoid the water being pushed back into the syringe.
- Attach the drainage bag and *gently* pull the catheter to ensure the inflated balloon sits at the neck of the bladder.
- If a residual catheter is used, remove the catheter once the bladder is emptied. These do not require drainage bags or the inflation of a balloon.
- Clear away the equipment and ensure the comfort of the woman. Wash hands.
- Measure and test the urine collected.

■ ALERT

No more than 1 litre of urine should be drained at any one time as this can result in shock.

■ FOLLOW-UP CARE AFTER INSERTION OF CATHETER

- Document actions in the woman's records and on the fluid balance chart. Especially note the amount of water inserted into the balloon.
- Attach the drainage bag to the stand. Ensure that the catheter never touches the floor and remains at a level below the bladder.
- Explain the care of the catheter to the woman; assist with putting underwear back on if needed.
- Ensure that vulval hygiene is maintained.

■ REMOVAL

- Ensure the woman's comfort and privacy.
- Wash hands and apply gloves. Use an apron.
- Deflate the balloon by withdrawing the water with a 10ml syringe. Explain to the woman that she may feel only some mild discomfort if anything.
- Withdraw the catheter gently.
- Empty and measure/test any urine remaining in the drainage bag.
- Dispose of the equipment, gloves and apron and wash hands.

■ FOLLOW-UP CARE AFTER REMOVAL

- Document the time of removal.
- Encourage the woman to drink clear fluids; inform her that she may feel some initial urgency to void urine due to urethral irritability.
- Note the time of the first void following removal to ensure that bladder function is unaffected. If unable to void urine within four hours refer to the medical team.

Cord bloods

Blood will be taken from the umbilical cord after the delivery of the placenta, for two main reasons:

1. Direct Coomb's – taken alongside a sample of the mother's blood to test for maternal antibodies in the fetal circulation. If present these could potentially lead to rhesus incompatibility, resulting in pathological jaundice. Only a sample of blood from the umbilical vein is required here. Maternal blood is sent for the Kleihauer test.
2. Blood samples from the vein and artery may be taken using pre-heparinised syringes to assess the degree of acidosis in the fetal blood. These are usually taken after an instrumental birth and after any suspected fetal compromise during a labour.

Notes

- A pH above 7.25 is normal. Below this suggests that some fetal acidosis has occurred.
- Respiratory acidosis is due to a buildup of CO_2 and a drop in oxygen levels. Usually aerobic metabolism can continue. However, metabolic acidosis occurs when the level of oxygen continues to fall. A resulting buildup of lactic acid leads to a high level of hydrogen ions which need buffers to be absorbed. As the buffers are used up the degree of acidosis increases. The greater the amount of buffers used the higher the base deficit.
- Therefore if metabolic respiration has occurred there is more likely to be a higher base excess reading as well as a low pH.

NB: Care must be taken to prevent any air bubbles from occurring in the samples, as this will alter the result.

Cord clamping

Historically, if conducting active management of the third stage of labour, the umbilical cord would be clamped and cut immediately following delivery of the baby. Current practice as recommended by NICE is to delay clamping the cord for between 1–5 minutes unless there is a clinical reason to do so such as if the baby requires transfer for resuscitation or the placenta needs to be delivered due to maternal haemorrhage. Delaying cord clamping enables the baby to receive valuable blood flow which can reduce risks of anaemia and iron deficiency resulting in affected growth and development. If left, the cord will naturally shut down and blood flow will cease (McDonald and Middleton 2009).

CTG interpretation

There are various ways of interpreting a cardiotocograph trace; however, they all consider the same components. The following (DrCBravado) is only one way. The key thing is to apply the physiology of the fetal CNS and circulatory system.

REMEMBER: Always check that the time and date are correct on the machine/trace and that the toco paddle is set at 20mmHg, which is the normal uterine resting pressure.

Dr = determine risk – consider the woman's pregnancy and medical history. Is she considered low, medium or high risk, and why?

C = contractions – consider the frequency (how many in a 10-minute period?), strength (on palpation) and regularity. Is there a resting gap between them or is there coupling?

Br = baseline rate – the mean level of the fetal heart rate, excluding accelerations and decelerations. Normal range 110–160bpm. Deviations can be caused by gestation, maternal pyrexia and tachycardia, and some drugs.

A = accelerations – increases above the baseline of 15bpm or more lasting 15 seconds or more.

Va = variability – the fluctuations from the baseline: should be greater than 5bpm. This is demonstrating that the parasympathetic and sympathetic nervous systems are working correctly.

D = decelerations – decreases from the baseline of 15bpm or more lasting 15 seconds or more.

- *Early* – uniform and repetitive. Onset early in the contraction and returns to baseline. Occurs in second stage due to head compression.
- *Variable* – vary in duration, frequency and usually have a rapid recovery to baseline. Can occur at any time, caused by cord compression. Shouldering is a positive sign.
- *Late* – uniform and repetitive. The peak occurs after the peak of the contraction. Caused by a delay in placental perfusion.
- *Prolonged deceleration* – an abrupt decrease in the heart rate lasting 60 seconds or more.

O = overall assessment and plan – is the CTG:
- *Normal* – are all the main features reassuring? Ask yourself: does it need to continue?
- *Suspicious* – are there any non-reassuring features (e.g. reduced variability)?
- *Pathological* – is more than one feature non-reassuring?

The management of these women is dependent on the overall picture and severity of any non-reassuring features.
    Possible options include any or all of the following:
- Alter maternal position – left lateral is often very effective.
- Check maternal observations. A sudden drop in BP (e.g. after an epidural top-up or ARM) can induce a prolonged deceleration.
- Refer to obstetric team and inform shift coordinator.
- Fetal blood sampling (FBS). NB: a drop in fetal blood pH and increase in base excess is significant. FBS may be performed more than once.
- Delivery.

Diabetic women in labour

Review both NICE (2015), RCOG and Trust guidelines to ensure you provide the best individualised care.

Routine labour care as for any woman plus:

- Review by obstetricians and diabetic specialists.
- Continuous fetal monitoring is recommended.
- Consider use of epidural for analgesia, especially if labour is augmented with oxytocin.
- Baseline bloods for FBC, urea and electrolytes (U&Es), group and save (G&S) and blood glucose. If hypertensive/pre-eclamptic also then a clotting screen may be required.
- Hourly capillary blood sugars using a recently calibrated monitor. Aim for readings between 4–7mmols/L.
- Test all urine for glucose and ketones.
- May commence an infusion of short-acting insulin mixed with normal saline via a pump. Sliding-scale insulin will be given adjusted according to the hourly blood sugar readings.
- If on sliding scale insulin commence a glucose 5% infusion (+/– KCL) via a pump.
- Clear fluids orally only.
- If an infusion of oxytocin is commenced, use a non-return valve giving set or a third cannula.
- *LABEL* all lines clearly when possible to avoid errors.
- Higher risk of shoulder dystocia, so be prepared!

NB: If steroids have recently been administered this can markedly affect the blood sugar levels.

Additional care will depend very much on the severity of the diabetes and how it has been managed.

■ AFTER BIRTH

- If gestational diabetes – discontinue the infusions once tolerating a light diet.
- If type 1 or type 2 – reduce the sliding scale as per policy and until tolerating diet.
- Administer a prescribed dose of subcutaneous (SC) insulin overlapping the end of the infusion by 30 minutes.
- Monitor blood sugars regularly at least pre-meal and pre-bed.
- Review by diabetic specialist to prescribe insulin regime/care management.
- Continue care on delivery suite until stabilised.
- Baby is also likely to need regular blood glucose monitoring.

External cephalic version (ECV)

This procedure is offered to women usually at between 36–38 weeks' gestation if their fetus is breech presentation at 36 weeks. With the additional risks associated with breech vaginal births, one way of reducing the need for a caesarean section is to turn the fetus into a cephalic presentation and aim for a normal labour and birth with less associated risks. It is suggested that 50–70% are successful. Some babies move back into the breech position. Rarely, the procedure can lead to the need for an urgent caesarean due to fetal distress or placental abruption during the procedure.

ECV involves the manipulation of the fetus by applying pressure to the fetus through the mother's abdomen. The aim is to push the fetus into a forward somersault (RCOG 2010).

■ PROCEDURE

- Explain and obtain informed consent.
- Ensure the woman's bladder is empty and she is comfortable in a semi-recumbent position.
- She may be asked to wear a hospital gown.
- Commonly a CTG is conducted prior to and after the procedure.
- The woman may be administered a uterine muscle relaxant such as Salbutamol or Tubertaline.
- A scan will be needed before and after to check fetal lie and presentation.
- The obstetrician will apply pressure to try to turn the fetus. Sometimes some powder may be needed to protect the mother's skin and aid grip.

- Once completed, the management will depend on the success of the ECV.
- Anti D may be prescribed if the mother is rhesus negative.
- Inform the woman of the outcome and subsequent management as well as signs of any issues which will require review, such as PV bleeding or reduced fetal movements.

This procedure can be quite uncomfortable for the woman and she will need your support and reassurance throughout. If all is successful she may be sent home, but not until there are no signs of any complications and follow-up is arranged.

Emergencies

■ SHOULDER DYSTOCIA

Where the anterior shoulder of the fetus becomes stuck behind the pubic bone of the pelvis. More common with large babies/macrosomia.

Figure 5 Managing shoulder dystocia

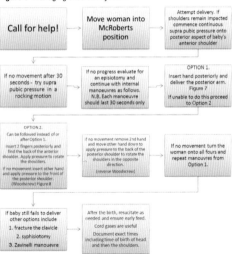

Figure 6 Delivery of the posterior arm

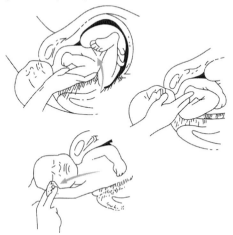

Figure 7 Woodscrew manoeuvre

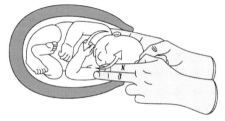

■ POST-PARTUM HAEMORRHAGE

Blood loss from the genital tract of 500ml or more or an amount which compromises the woman following the birth. Primary within 24 hours and secondary 24 hours to 6 weeks postnatal.

Figure 8 Management of post-partum haemorrhage

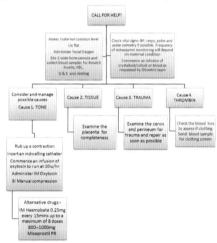

If bleeding persists transfer to theatre. Can try a Blynch suture, ballon tamponade, artery embolisation, hysterectomy.

REMEMBER to estimate the overall blood loss (including weighing pads, etc.) and document all events.

After care should include:

- HDU/DS/ward.
- Regular MEOWS monitoring alongside antiembolic stockings and VTE scoring.
- Repeat bloods for Hb and treat any deficiency.
- Assist with baby, especially if breastfeeding and anaemic.
- Debrief.

■ NEONATAL RESUSCITATION

Figure 9 Neonatal resuscitation

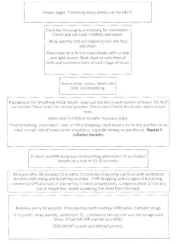

Source: Adapted from Resuscitation Council UK (2019).

■ BREECH

Breech birth. Where the buttocks are presenting at the brim of the pelvis. Baby can have extended legs, flexed legs, or can present with a foot or knee on one or both legs.

Figure 10 Breech delivery

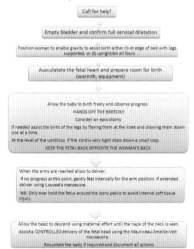

■ CORD PROLAPSE

Where the cord precedes the presenting part following a rupture of membranes. Cord presentation my be present prior to any rupture of membranes.

Figure 11 Cord prolapse

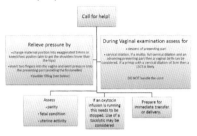

Call for help!

Relieve pressure by
• change maternal position into exaggerated Sims or knee/chest position (aim to get the shoulders lower than the hips)
• insert two fingers into the vagina and exert pressure onto the presenting part (avoiding the fontanelles)
• bladder filling (see below)

During Vaginal examination assess for
• descent of presenting part
• cervical dilation. If a multip, full cervical dilation and an advancing presenting part then a vaginal birth can be considered. If a primip with a cervical dilation of 3cm then a LSCS is likely.

DO NOT handle the cord

Assess
• parity
• fetal condition
• uterine activity

If an oxytocin infusion is running this needs to be stopped. Use of a tocolytic may be considered

Prepare for immediate transfer or delivery.

■ BLADDER FILLING

If successful, filling the woman's bladder can raise the presenting part out of the pelvis and off the cord by up to 2cm, which allows time for transfer to a unit from the community or to prepare for delivery in a more controlled way.
- Gain consent.
- Cleanse vulva if able.
- Insert an indwelling catheter and empty the bladder of urine. Inflate the balloon.
- Insert the end of an intravenous infusion giving set into the end of the catheter (where the bag is normally inserted) and infuse up to 700ml of room temperature normal saline into the bladder. Clamp the catheter and detach the giving set. If this action successfully raises the presenting part, the fingers can be removed from the vagina. If unsuccessful, digital pressure must continue until delivery.
- If a LSCS is undertaken the bladder must be emptied prior to the first incision.

Emergency birth

Women can give birth at anytime and anywhere, so it is useful to give some thought as to how you would deal with a birth outside of the home or a maternity unit.

Here are some tips. Think about:

- **What information do I need?** Name, gestation, parity, number of babies, any obstetric/medical history.
- **What's happening?** Think = contractions, stage of labour, any sign of the presenting part.
- **What do I do first?** Get help, health and safety, privacy, support.
- **What equipment do I need?** Some protection for hands (e.g. clean plastic bags), towels/something to dry and wrap the baby in.
- **What do I do with the baby?** If birth progresses normally and the baby is in good condition – note time of birth, dry the baby and wrap to keep warm – preferably commence skin-to-skin with mother. If baby is compromised, then initiate basic life support.
- **What do I do with the placenta/third stage?** Don't worry about clamping and cutting the cord (the cord should clamp itself naturally). If the mother and baby are stable leave well alone. If the placenta delivers, put it into a bag or some kind of container to transfer with the mother to the unit for examination.

Epidurals

An epidural can be sited at any point during established labour as long as the anaesthetist is able to carry out the procedure and the woman is able to maintain the required position for long enough. It is also possible that an epidural could be sited prior to the commencement of an oxytocin infusion for induction of labour, although in these cases it can be very difficult to ascertain whether the epidural is working effectively until contractions are occurring. It is also recommended that women with high BMIs have an anaesthetic review during the antenatal period and have an epidural sited early.

■ ADVANTAGES OF AN EPIDURAL

- Can provide complete pain relief.
- If there is any likelihood of the need for a Caesarean or assisted birth the route for an anaesthetic is already *in situ*.
- Can help women relax and cope with their labour, especially if having persistent back pain.
- Can lower blood pressure which can be beneficial in women with pre-eclampsia.
- Useful for reducing stress in women with cardiac disease.

■ DISADVANTAGES OF AN EPIDURAL

- Will reduce mobility which can slow the progress of labour.
- The sensation to micturate may be lost, increasing the need for a catheter.
- There may be segments of the abdomen that are not anaesthetised.

- Women with infections, pyrexia, clotting disorders or a very high body mass index (BMI) may not be suitable to receive an epidural.
- There is likely to be a need to have continuous fetal monitoring – increasing the problems associated with reduced mobility.
- Risk of complications such as a persistent headache or dural tap.
- Increased risk of thrombosis, pressure sores due to reduced mobility.
- Can increase the incidence of instrumental birth.
- Women may not like the sensation.

■ PROCEDURE

- Ideally, discussion around pain relief should have occurred prior to labour starting, but, if not, the procedure, benefits and disadvantages must be shared. The anaesthetist is also required to do this when obtaining consent. The anaesthetist must be informed if the woman has been on any low molecular weight heparin for any reason.
- Ensure that the woman has emptied her bladder prior to starting the procedure.
- A wide-bore cannula will be sited and a loading dose of around 500ml fluid administered (commonly Hartmann's solution). This is to minimise the impact of a likely drop in blood pressure after the first dose of anaesthetic.
- As the cannula is sited it is an ideal time to take blood samples for at least a group and save and a full blood count.
- Ideally the fetal heart rate should be monitored throughout the procedure, although this can sometimes be difficult due to maternal position.

- A baseline blood pressure and pulse should be taken and recorded.
- The woman will be sat on the edge of the bed with her feet on a stool in a curled-up position. Pillows can be helpful to rest her head and arms on. Alternatively, she will be asked to adopt the fetal position on her left side with her knees drawn up and her chin tucked in. Either position enables better access to the spaces between the vertebrae. The anaesthetist will opt for one of these positions, but if there is suspected fetal compromise then the left lateral position is optimal.
- The equipment (see Figure 12) needs to be set up on a clean trolley and the anaesthetist will need to wear a mask, sterile gown and gloves. The gown will need to be tied at the back by a helper.
- The woman's back will be cleansed with antiseptic lotion and the site for the epidural identified. The area will be injected with local anaesthetic. Once the area is numb, the anaesthetist will insert the epidural and when happy inject a test dose of anaesthetic (e.g. Bupivacaine).
- While this is taking effect, the epidural catheter will be taped in place and the woman's position may be changed to encourage the anaesthetic to spread to all areas of the abdomen.
- The blood pressure must be taken every 5 minutes for at least 20 minutes with the test and any subsequent top-up doses of anaesthetic.
- The anaesthetist should complete an epidural chart and the procedure and drugs administered should be accurately recorded.

Epidural equipment

Figure 12 Epidural equipment

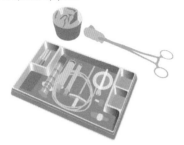

■ CARE OF A WOMAN WITH AN EPIDURAL *IN SITU*

NB: This will largely depend on Trust policy, but here are some pointers:

- Blood pressure should be taken at least every hour.
- Fetal well-being should be continuously monitored (unless policy states exclusion criteria for this).
- Either an indwelling catheter or residual catheters may be used. If not, encourage the use of bedpans or if a mobile epidural is administered encourage mobility to the toilet.
- Change maternal position as often as possible.
- Ensure the bed is clean and pads are changed regularly.
- Drugs such as Ranitidine 150mg every 6 hours may be prescribed.

- There is likely to be a physiological rise in temperature which is common – therefore take temperature at least hourly. Report any deviations from a normal temperature. Paracetamol can be an effective way of reducing a temperature.
- Monitor the level of block (training for this is needed) and also monitor the woman's well-being – symptoms such as tingling in the fingers or lips or breathlessness should be reported immediately.
- If the woman has a raised BMI as well – apply elastic support stockings and consider manual handling issues.
- **Do not** let the pain relief wear off, not even in the second stage to aid pushing.
- It can be beneficial, if there is no evidence of fetal compromise and the contractions are strong and regular, to delay the commencement of active pushing from the onset of the second stage of labour for around an hour. This enables the contractions to push the fetus down the birth canal and reduces the time the woman has to push. Evidence suggests that this lessens the likelihood of an instrumental birth (see Anim-Somuah, Smyth and Howell 2005).
- After the birth – remove the epidural cannula unless instructed otherwise. Examine the end to ensure that it is complete. Apply a sterile dressing to the site which must remain *in situ* for a minimum of 24 hours.
- Women should not get out of bed until full feeling in their legs has returned. It is also vital to check bladder function following birth and to help the woman care for her baby, as she will be restricted until full mobility returns.

Episiotomy

A surgical incision of the perineum used to expedite birth. Reasons include instrumental birth, breech, shoulder dystocia if internal manoeuvres are used, female genital mutilation (FGM) and fetal distress. Little evidence supports routine episiotomy for premature births or previous third- or fourth-degree tears.

■ PROCEDURE

- Gain consent.
- With two fingers inserted to protect the fetus, infiltrate the perineum with up to 10ml local anaesthetic (e.g. lidocaine 1%). This should be done when the perineum is not stretched by pressure from the presenting part.
- Insert the episiotomy scissors, continuing to protect the fetus with two fingers inserted.
- At the point when the perineum is fully stretched, perform a single clean cut laterally from the fourchette (imagine the direction of number seven on a clock face).
- Bleeding is likely; therefore keep the area covered with clean pads when possible. Avoid contamination with faecal matter.
- Repair of the trauma should be completed as quickly as possible after the birth to minimise blood loss.
- Educate the woman about care of the perineum and document actions.

TIP

If you are left-handed you might need to change the side of the bed you are working to achieve the correct angle.

Examination of the placenta

It is vital that the placenta and membranes are examined after every delivery. If there is any suspicion that they are incomplete, then staff must be extra vigilant when monitoring the mother's well-being as she is more at risk of experiencing a post-partum haemorrhage.

- Examine the placenta on a flat surface.
- Examine the maternal side first – check that all of the cotyledons are present. Are there any gaps or extra lobes? Note the condition and colour of the tissue. A gritty placenta can suggest that the mother smokes. Are there any large clots of blood on this surface (retroplacental clots)? These can suggest that an abruption has occurred.
- Examine the fetal surface. Lay the membranes out and check for holes. Quite often the membranes are ragged which should be clearly documented. Peel the membranes apart to check that there are two.
- Check the cord. There should be two small arteries and a larger vein. Check the length of cord for any true knots.
- Take any cord bloods if needed.
- Carefully dispose of the placenta as per Trust policy.
- Document your findings.

Fetal blood sampling

■ EQUIPMENT

- Vaginal examination or FBS pack – blade holder, capillary tube holder, amniscope, forceps, gauze swabs.
- Obstetric cream and paraffin jelly.
- Light source.
- Ethyl Chloride spray.
- Blood gas machine.
- Capillary tubes and ends.
- Cleansing lotion.

■ PROCEDURE

- Obtain consent.
- Position woman in left lateral or lithotomy.
- Cleanse the vulva and insert the amniscope.
- Attach light source and, once visualised, the presenting part will be wiped.
- Spray Ethyl Chloride onto presenting part.
- The obstetrician will make a small incision and draw up samples using the capillary tubes. Plug off the ends of the tubes and transfer to the blood gas machine for analysis.

The management will depend on the result. Labour will be allowed to continue without further tests; or a repeat test in 30–60 minutes; or urgent delivery may be required.

Home birth preparation

Home birth can be considered as safe as a hospital birth as long as there is adequate preparation.

Aspects to consider include:

Education – ensure the woman and the staff are prepared.

Safety – make sure that there aren't any domestic violence or child protection issues which could place staff in danger.

Support – make sure there is adequate support from colleagues.

The family – it is the woman's home and she can have whoever she wishes present.

The environment – e.g. is there enough room? Remember health and safety and manual handling for the staff as well as for the woman. Also is there adequate heating?

Hygiene – is the environment as clean as possible? Is there access to hand-washing facilities?

Accessibility – if the need arose, can the location be easily accessed by emergency services and the woman transferred safely?

Initial baby check

This top-to-toe examination should be conducted in a warm, draught-free, well-lit environment and in the presence of the parents. Consent should be obtained.

- Wash hands and apply clean gloves.
  NB: Only expose the area you are examining to avoid the baby losing heat.
- Check the overall condition of the skin – any rashes, trauma.
- Consider the baby's overall tone, colour and alertness.
- Head – check the shape, trauma (bruising, etc.); fontanelles (these should not be bulging or sunken); position and clarity of eyes; position and patency of ears; nose is shaped normally and has two patent nostrils.
- Mouth – examine the mouth for any abnormalities (e.g. teeth, harelip, tongue ties). To check that the palate is completely formed, a tongue depressor and light source are considered optimal.
- Check the neck for any webbing.
- Examine the chest and abdomen – there should be two nipples, evenly spaced. The chest should be rising evenly. Count the baby's respirations if needed. The abdomen should be soft and rounded. The cord should be securely clamped.
- Arms – check they are of equal length and shape. Check the hands – the number of palmar creases, digits, is there any webbing between the fingers?

- Examine the genitalia – females: check there are labia, urethral and vaginal orifice. Female infants may pass a small amount of blood or have a clear discharge – this is normal. Males: check there is a patent urethral opening at the end of the penis – rule out any hypospadias and feel for two testes within the scrotal sac. The anus should be patent. Document that female genitalia is intact in line with recommendations for reducing FGM.
- Legs – check there are two of equal length and shape. Examine the feet for talipes or webbing between the toes. Count the toes.
- Turn the baby over and examine the spine for any dimples or abnormalities (e.g. Mongolian blue spot).
- Measure the head circumference (and length, if local policy, from the occiput to the heel of the foot).
- Weigh the baby.
- If not already done – take the baby's temperature (normal = 36.5°C–37.2°C).
- Apply two identity labels and if policy a security tag.
- Administer vitamin K if requested.
- Dress the baby or continue with skin-to-skin.
- Feed the baby as soon as possible.
- Document findings.

Instrumental birth

Types include ventouse/kiwi cup.

Figure 13 A kiwi cup

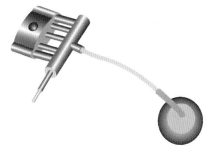

Forceps types (e.g. Wrigley's (low cavity); Neville-Barnes (mid-cavity) and Keilland's (rotational)).

Figure 14 Wrigley's forceps

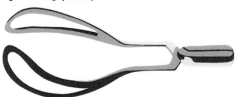

■ PREPARATION

- Establish the reason for the procedure and the method to be used.
- Gain consent from the mother (bear in mind that this is usually an emergency situation, so explanations may be quite brief).
- Call for help – extra midwives and a paediatrician.
- Ensure adequate analgesia – top up the epidural if time, or provide the equipment for a pudendal block and lidocaine 1% for perineal infiltration.
- Assist the woman into the lithotomy position – remove end of bed.
- Ensure the fetal heart is monitored – preferably by CTG.
- Open the forceps pack and provide the appropriate equipment for the obstetrician (catheter, forceps or ventouse, obstetric cream, cleansing lotion, suturing equipment).
- The vulva should be cleansed and the bladder emptied.
- Reassure the woman and partner as often as possible. Explain what is happening.
- Once the instruments have been applied, palpate for contractions and encourage pushing during these.
- Active third stage is encouraged following an instrumental birth due to the higher risk of post-partum haemorrhage (PPH); therefore once the baby is born the administration of an oxytocin is recommended.
- Provide assistance with any required resuscitation of the baby.
- Once the procedure is completed ensure the woman's comfort and document the events.

Mechanism of normal labour (LOA)

- The widest presenting diameter enters the widest diameter of the brim (transverse) of the pelvis.
- The head will flex during engagement at the brim to present the suboccipito-bregmatic (SOB) diameter (9.5cm) of the vertex.
- **Descent** through the pelvis is aided by pressure exerted by regular strong uterine contractions.
- **Flexion and fetal axis pressure** – when the head meets the resistance of the birth canal and pressure is directed down the body of the fetus onto the occiput, further flexion occurs.
- The occiput meets the resistance of the pelvic floor, causing **internal rotation** of the head one-eighth of a circle anteriorly.
- The occiput escapes under the pubic arch and **crowning** occurs.
- **Extension** takes place where the forehead and face sweep the perineum.
- **Restitution** – the neck untwists to line up the head and shoulders again.
- **Internal rotation of the shoulders and external rotation of the head** occurs to line the shoulders up into the anterior posterior diameter of the pelvic outlet.
- **Lateral flexion** – the anterior shoulder is usually released under the pubic arch first followed by the posterior shoulder (this may alter depending on maternal position at birth). This movement may be aided by the midwife.
- **Expulsion** – the baby's body is born.

Monitoring maternal and fetal well-being in labour

- At the start of labour or at any change-over of staff, a review of the medical and obstetric history should be undertaken.
- A baseline set of observations are required – BP, pulse, respirations, temperature and urinalysis.
- The frequency of repeating these observations will depend on Trust policy and maternal condition – commonly BP = hourly, pulse every 30 minutes, temperature every 4 hours.
- All urine output should be measured and tested for ketones, protein and glucose.
- A baseline abdominal examination should be undertaken and repeated prior to any vaginal examinations or used as an alternative to assess progress in labour.
- Women should be encouraged to empty their bladder every two hours.
- Dependent on risk status and stage of labour, women may eat light meals for energy and drink fluids to maintain hydration.
- Analgesia as required.
- Support and reassurance.
- Information and feedback at every step.
- Documentation.
- Assessment of progress – clinical signs or using vaginal examination (commonly 3–4 hourly).
- Monitor strength and frequency of contractions – don't rely on the tocograph. Palpation provides more information.

- Fetal monitoring – NICE (2019b) recommend an assessment every 15 minutes in the first stage of labour for a full 60 seconds and after each contraction or every 5 minutes during the second stage. A pinard stethoscope *must* be used where possible unless a CTG is in progress which must be reviewed every 15 minutes.
- Assessment of vaginal loss – any bleeding or meconium should be reported.
- Preparation of the environment and equipment.
- Encourage use of birth equipment, and different positions to promote contractions (Gupta and Nikodem 2002).
- Administer any oxytocic drug for active third-stage management if chosen.

Additional care may include:

- Inserting a cannula and taking baseline blood tests.
- Insertion of an indwelling catheter.
- Administration of antacids (e.g. Ranitidine 150mg orally).
- Administer antibiotics for prolonged ruptured membranes or known Group B Streptococcus infection.
- Perform an artificial rupture of membranes, apply a fetal scalp electrode.

Obesity and labour

Women with a high BMI in labour still need the routine care that any woman in labour requires. However, there are a few extra considerations:

- Due to the greater risk, these women should give birth under consultant-led care.
- Obesity itself is not an indication for induction of labour.
- Early assessment by the anaesthetist and obstetrician (prior to labour preferably) is optimal.
- If requested, the insertion of an epidural by a senior anaesthetist earlier in the labour is preferable. However, the benefits of encouraging mobility to promote normal labour and reduce the risks of thrombosis should also be considered.
- Equipment, including beds and birthing balls, blood pressure cuffs, etc., should be capable of accommodating the woman's weight.
- One-to-one continuous care is vital.
- Manual handling and health and safety issues must be considered. Use elastic support stockings if mobility is restricted.
- Venous access if BMI is over 40.
- Active management of the third stage is advocated.
- Continuous monitoring may be required but can be difficult; there may be a case for the use of a fetal scalp electrode (FSE).
- **Remember:** Women with a high BMI may have been on heparin during the antenatal period and so are at a higher risk of haemorrhage.
- There is an increased risk of shoulder dystocia, so consider adopting alternative positions for the birth where possible (CMACE/RCOG 2010; Rees et al. 2008).

Pain relief

The options for pain relief in labour are numerous and the decision as to which to use should be the woman's. Every individual will manage the discomfort of labour differently and may change their minds at any point as labour progresses. It is highly possible that more than one of the options listed below are selected. Other women, however, may opt to have a completely natural birth. The role of the midwife is therefore to support and guide the woman using appropriate information and administering where possible the method of choice.

■ NON-PHARMACOLOGICAL

NB: Those options indicated by an asterisk (*) require appropriate training to administer and may not be available at every unit. Not all of these options have scientific evidence to support their effectiveness, but anecdotal evidence suggests that they can be extremely beneficial for some women.

- Water.
- Relaxation.
- Massage.
- Hypnosis.*
- Aromatherapy.*
- Reflexology.*
- Acupuncture.*
- Yoga* and alternative positioning.
- Transcutaneous electrical nerve stimulation (TENS).

■ PHARMACOLOGICAL

- Nitrous oxide and oxygen (Entonox).
- Paracetamol/codydramol (in early labour).
- Pethidine or meptid.
- Morphine.
- Epidural.
- Spinal.
- Pudendal block (for instrumental births).
- Lidocaine/lignocaine 1% for infiltration prior to an episiotomy or perineal repair.

Perineal repair

Degrees of perineal trauma

Labial, clitoral lacerations/tears.

1st degree – skin +/– superficial vaginal wall.

2nd degree – skin, vaginal wall and muscle **(equates to an episiotomy).**

3rd degree – skin, vaginal wall, superficial and deep muscles and external anal sphincter.

4th degree – skin, vaginal wall, muscle layer, external and internal sphincter.

Process

- Position the woman in lithotomy position to enable good visability. Have a good light source.
- Inspect trauma. Third- or fourth-degree tears ***must*** be repaired by an obstetrician.
- Set up equipment and position yourself comfortably. Count the swabs, needles and instruments.
- Cleanse area with sterile lotion and apply sterile field/drapes.
- Infiltrate the wound with 10–20ml of local anaesthetic (e.g. Lidocaine 1%). Giving the woman Entonox is helpful here or top up the epidural.
- Insert a tampon if needed – secure tape end to drape.
- Insert an anchor stitch 1cm above the apex of the tear in the vaginal wall. Vicryl rapide 2.0 is a commonly recommended suture material.
- Repair vagina using a continuous non-locking stitch.

- Bring the needle beneath the hymenal ring into the muscle layer and continue the non-locking stitch to close the muscle layers.
- At the end, reverse the needle and repair the skin using a continuous subcuticular stitch.
- Insert the needle back into the vagina approximately 1cm behind the forchette and finish with a terminal loop knot.
- Inspect the repair for any gaps or bleeding points. Haemostasis should have occurred.
- Perform a rectal examination inserting PR analgesia (e.g. Diclofenac), if needed.
- Remove the tampon. Cleanse the area and apply a clean pad.
- Ensure the woman's comfort.
- Count the swabs, needles and instruments.
- Document.
- Educate the woman about hygiene – wash hands before and after toilet/changing pads (CMACE 2011).

Positions for labour and birth

Positions for first stage of labour

ACTIVITY

Think about how these positions may help birth, revisit the pelvis and mechanism of labour to help you. Are there any disadvantages?

Figure 15 Labour and birth positions

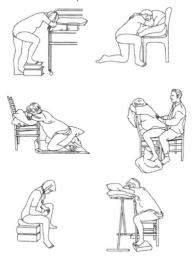

Resuscitation equipment

Neonatal bag and mask

Figure 16 Neonatal bag and mask

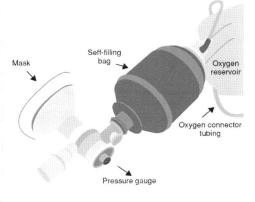

Mask

Seff-filling
bag

Oxygen
reservoir

Oxygen connector
tubing

Pressure gauge

SBAR handover

The SBAR tool has been designed to aid effective communication between professionals, especially during critical situations. The main principles to work to are:

- **S – SITUATION –** What is happening now?
- **B – BACKGROUND –** What has happened that is relevant to this situation?
- **A – ASSESSMENT –** In your view what is the problem/issue?
- **R – RECOMMENDATIONS –** What do you think needs to happen now? What actions do you propose?

Signs of transition

There are numerous signs and symptoms exhibited by a woman in the transition stage of labour. The following are some of the more common ones:

- The contractions slow and become less frequent prior to a change to more expulsive contractions. If the contractions slow or even stop and don't return, this must be referred to an obstetrician and/or the senior midwife.
- Vomiting.
- Maternal grunting.
- Urges to push (NB: these may be early if the fetus is in an occipito posterior position; however, the cervix may not be dilated to 10cm).
- Presenting part visible.
- Change in the woman's behaviour (may become angry, upset, express concerns of being unable to continue, etc.).
- Change of maternal position. Some women turn into a semi-recumbent position drawing their knees up, or become more upright.
- Heavy blood-stained show.
- Pouting anus or vulval gaping.
- Purple/red line at the cleft of the buttocks.
- Rhomboid of Michaelas (where the triangular-shaped sacrum is pushed backwards).

Stages and phases of labour

Latent phase The buildup prior to the active first stage
of labour which can last for a few days. During this time irregular niggles, backache and mild contractions occur. The
cervix also begins to soften and efface (flatten out from a
tube to a ring) and dilate. There may be a blood-streaked
mucousy show and possibly a spontaneous rupture of
membranes.

First stage From the onset of regular contractions (building
to 3–5 every 10 minutes, which last for up to 60 seconds),
accompanied by cervical dilatation from 4cm to the full
dilatation of the cervical os.

Transition phase Occurs between the end of the first stage
and the onset of the second stage of labour. See the Signs
of transition section (p. 55).

Second stage From full dilatation of the cervical os to the
birth of the baby.

Third stage From the birth of the baby to the birth of the
placenta and membranes and the control of bleeding.

Some midwives refer to the **fourth stage** of labour, which
includes the repair of the perineum.

Third-stage management

■ PHYSIOLOGICAL/EXPECTANT

- Can take up to 60 minutes.
- The placenta and membranes are expelled by maternal effort.
- **Do not** administer any oxytocin, palpate the uterus, apply cord traction or clamp and cut the cord.
- Observe for signs of separation – cord lengthening, small gush of blood PV, return of an urge to push, placenta visible.
- Assist the woman into an upright position and encourage pushing.
- Catch placenta and membranes in a bowl. The partner, mother or midwife can now clamp and cut the cord.

TIP

Encouraging skin-to-skin and/or breastfeeding will release natural oxytocin, which will aid contractions.

NB: If there is a need for neonatal or maternal resuscitation due to haemorrhage, changing to active management may be required.

■ ACTIVE

- 1 to 30 minutes.
- Aided by the administration of an oxytocic drug and controlled cord traction (CCT).

- Administer oxytocin into the mother's thigh coinciding with the birth of the baby's anterior shoulder or as soon as possible.
- Clamp and cut the cord. A 2–3-minute delay prior to this can prove beneficial unless the baby is born requiring resuscitation (see McDonald and Middleton 2009).
- Remember to clamp off a 10cm section of cord if cord gases are needed.
- Palpate the uterine fundus to check for separation (feels like a hard ball at about the umbilicus).
- Guarding the uterus with one hand, apply downward traction on the cord with the other. The traction should be continuous and smooth.
- If the placenta is not delivering **stop** CCT and retry after rechecking the fundus.
- As the placenta reaches the vulva continue with upward flexion.
- Collect the placenta in a bowl. If possible, contain the clots by gently twisting the membranes to form a bag around them.

TIP

Syntometrine® 1ml containing 500 micrograms of Ergometrine maleate and 5iu of oxytocin is commonly used for active third-stage management. However, as it causes vasoconstriction it should be avoided in women with hypertension.

Vaginal examination

- Before you start, make sure you have a good reason for undertaking the assessment. Ask yourself whether there is another way of assessing progress.
- You must obtain consent to perform the examination and document it.
- Perform an abdominal examination – this should support your findings from the VE.
- Prepare your equipment – VE pack, sterile/non-sterile gloves as appropriate, cleansing solution, lubricant. Have ready an amnihook or fetal scalp electrode if you are likely to need it.
- Position the woman comfortably.
- Ensure that dignity and privacy is maintained.
- Cleanse the vulva area and proceed with the examination.
- Undertake any additional tasks – artificial rupture of membrane (ARM), insertion of prostaglandin, or attach a fetal scalp electrode (FSE).
- On completion – ensure the comfort of the woman, explain your findings and document them.
- Undertake appropriate management as required.

■ DOCUMENTING A VAGINAL EXAMINATION

Remember to always palpate first and to assess fetal well-being afterwards.

- External genitalia (e.g. no abnormalities detected (NAD), FGM).
- Vagina – moist, dry and hot, NAD.
- Cervix:
  - position – central, anterior, posterior, lateral
  - consistency – soft, firm
  - effacement – fully effaced, thick, thin

- application – well applied, loosely applied
- dilatation – 1 to 10cm, anterior rim.
- Membranes – absent, intact.
- Liquor – meconium, clear, blood-stained.
- Presenting part:
  - confirm cephalic, breech, shoulder
  - exclude cord presentation
  - station to ischial spines −3 to +2
  - identify landmarks and position (e.g. left occipito-anterior (LOA), occipito-posterior (OP)).

Figure 17 Station of presenting part

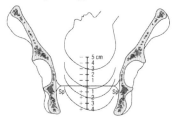

TIP

You don't have to get a woman into the semi-recumbent position to examine her. Try alternatives.

TIP

If she is semi-recumbent and you cannot reach the cervix, try putting something under the woman's buttocks to tilt her pelvis upward (e.g. asking the woman to put her clenched fists underneath her bottom works well).

Vaginal birth after Caesarean (VBAC)

Around 75% of VBAC women will have a successful vaginal birth after CS within a hospital or home environment; some even have pool births. Occasionally, the reason for a repeat CS in the remaining 25% is uterine rupture; however, the risks still exist (Horn 2003).

Caution must be taken when considering ARM, induction and/or augmentation with oxytocic drugs (Chapman 2018).

Routine care plus:

- In hospital continuous fetal monitoring is expected. Otherwise diligent intermittent auscultation.
- Large-bore cannula – dependent on the woman's choice, location and policy.
- Baseline bloods for FBC and group and save.
- 6-hourly antacids/hydrogen ion inhibitors (e.g. Ranitidine 150mg).
- Analgesia – an epidural is often recommended but is not compulsory.
- If aiming for a home birth – plan in advance how an emergency would be dealt with.

Signs of rupture

- PAIN – sudden onset, especially in lower abdomen or over scar area. May get no relief from any epidural top-ups.
- CONTRACTIONS – continuous or stop completely. Uterus becomes hard and rigid.
- FETAL HEART – variable and/or late decelerations or a sudden prolonged bradycardia.

- WOMAN – agitation and restlessness; altered vital signs.
- BLEEDING – fresh bleeding per vagina or blood-stained liquor.

TIP

If in any doubt get reviewed by senior staff/transferred immediately.

Waterbirth

Routine care in labour plus:

- One-to-one care is necessary – never leave a woman alone when she is using the pool.
- Remember to have training in using the pool and dealing with any emergencies that may occur.
- Remember manual handling issues and your personal health and safety.
- Check the woman's temperature hourly.
- Encourage the intake of fluids as dieresis increases when in water.
- Test the water temperature every 30 minutes and adjust to between 35 and 37°C.
- Abdominal and vaginal assessments can be carried out in the pool.
- Fetal heart monitoring can be intermittent using a waterproof Doppler device or using telemetry continuous monitoring if available.
- For the second stage the water temperature should be maintained at 37°C.
- A mirror can be used to view progress.
- Hands off the birth unless assistance is deemed necessary!
- The woman can raise the baby to the surface herself or the midwife can do so.
- Assess the baby's condition but remember that these babies don't often cry straight away.
- Avoid putting the baby back under the water once the head is above the surface.

- The third stage can be conducted either in the pool or on dry land.
- Allow approximately 1 hour, unless there is excessive bleeding, before any perineal repair to allow the tissues to become less waterlogged (Garland 2011).

References

ANIM-SOMUAH, M., SMYTH, R. D. and HOWELL, C. J. (2005) *Epidural versus Non-epidural or no Analgesia in Labour.* www.cochrane.org.

CHAPMAN, V. Charles C. (2018) *The Midwife's Labour and Birth Handbook* (4th edition). Oxford: Blackwell.

CMACE (2011) *Saving Mothers' Lives.* London: BJOG.

CMACE/RCOG (2010) *Management of Women with Obesity in Pregnancy.* London: Centre for Maternal and Child Enquiries and the RCOG.

GARLAND, D. (2011) *Revisiting Waterbirth. An Attitude to Care.* Basingstoke: Palgrave Macmillan.

GUPTA, J. K. and NIKODEM, V. C. (2002) *Woman's Position during the Second Stage of Labour.* Cochrane Review. The Cochrane Library, issue 4. Oxford: Update Software.

HORN, A. (2003) *VBAC at Home.* www.homebirth.org.uk.

McDONALD, S. J. and MIDDLETON, P. (2009) *Effect of Timing of Umbilical Cord Clamping at Birth in Term Infants on Mother and Baby Outcomes.* www.cochrane.org.

NATIONAL INSTITUTE for HEALTH and CARE EXCELLENCE (2015) *Diabetes in Pregnancy. Management from Preconception to the Postnatal Period.* NG3. London: NICE.

NATIONAL INSTITUTE for HEALTH and CARE EXCELLENCE (2019a) *Caesarean Section.* London: NICE.

NATIONAL INSTITUTE for HEALTH and CARE EXCELLENCE (2019b) *Intrapartum Care.* London: NICE.

REES, M., KANOSHI, M. and KEITH, L. (eds) (2008) *Obesity and Pregnancy.* London: Royal Society of Medicine Press.

RESUSCIATION COUNCIL UK (2019) *Resuscitation Guidelines*. London: Resuscitation Council UK.

ROYAL COLLEGE of MIDWIVES (2018) *Midwifery Care in Labour Guidance for all Women in all Settings. Blue Top Guideline no 1*. www.rcm.org.uk.

ROYAL COLLEGE of OBSTETRICIANS and GYNAECOLOGISTS (2010) *Externa Cephalic Version and Reducing the Incidence of Breech Presentation. Guideline 20A*. London: RCOG.

Student Notes